I0482998

Reference Information

Individuals who wish to cite this statement should use the following format:

Cunningham FG, Bangdiwala S, Brown SS, Dean TM, Frederiksen M, Rowland Hogue CJ, King T, Spencer Lukacz E, McCullough LB, Nicholson W, Petit N, Probstfield JL, Viguera AC, Wong CA, Zimmet SC. National Institutes of Health Consensus Development Conference Statement: Vaginal Birth After Cesarean: New Insights. March 8–10, 2010. Obstetrics & Gynecology. 2010; 115(6):1279–1295.

Publications Ordering Information

NIH Consensus Statements, State-of-the-Science Statements, and related materials are available by visiting ***http://consensus.nih.gov***; by calling toll free **888–644–2667**; or by emailing ***consensus@mail.nih.gov***. Written requests can be mailed to the NIH Consensus Development Program Information Center, P.O. Box 2577, Kensington, MD 20891. When ordering copies of this statement, please reference item number **2010-00122-STMT**.

The evidence report prepared for this conference through AHRQ is available on the web via ***http://www.ahrq.gov/clinic/tp/vbacuptp.htm***. Printed copies may be ordered from the AHRQ Publications Clearinghouse by calling **800–358–9295**. Requesters should ask for AHRQ Publication No. **10-E003**.

NIH Consensus Development Conference Statement on

Vaginal Birth After Cesarean: New Insights

NIH Consensus and State-of-the-Science Statements

Volume 27, Number 3
March 8–10, 2010

NATIONAL INSTITUTES OF HEALTH
Office of the Director

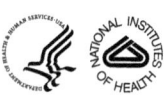

Archived Conference Webcast

The NIH Consensus Development Conference on Vaginal Birth After Cesarean: New Insights was webcast live March 8–10, 2010. The webcast is archived and available for viewing free of charge at *http://consensus.nih.gov/2010/vbac.htm*.

Abstract

Objective

To provide healthcare providers, patients, and the general public with a responsible assessment of currently available data on vaginal birth after cesarean (VBAC).

Participants

A non-Department of Health and Human Services, nonadvocate 15-member panel representing the fields of obstetrics and gynecology, urogynecology, maternal and fetal medicine, pediatrics, midwifery, clinical pharmacology, medical ethics, internal medicine, family medicine, perinatal and reproductive psychiatry, anesthesiology, nursing, biostatistics, epidemiology, healthcare regulation, risk management, and a public representative. In addition, 20 experts from pertinent fields presented data to the panel and conference audience.

Evidence

Presentations by experts and a systematic review of the literature prepared by the Oregon Evidence-based Practice Center, through the Agency for Healthcare Research and Quality (AHRQ). Scientific evidence was given precedence over anecdotal experience.

Conference Process

The panel drafted its statement based on scientific evidence presented in open forum and on published scientific literature. The draft statement was presented on the final day of the conference and circulated to the audience for comment. The panel released a revised statement later that day at *http://consensus.nih.gov*. This statement is an independent report of the panel and is not a policy statement of the National Institutes of Health (NIH) or the Federal Government.

Conclusions

Given the available evidence, trial of labor is a reasonable option for many pregnant women with one prior low transverse uterine incision. The data reviewed in this report show that both trial of labor and elective repeat cesarean delivery for a pregnant woman with one prior transverse uterine incision have important risks and benefits and that these risks and benefits differ for the woman and her fetus. This poses a profound ethical dilemma for the woman, as well as her caregivers, because benefit for the woman may come at the price of increased risk for the fetus and vice versa. This conundrum is worsened by the general paucity of high-level evidence about both medical and nonmedical factors, which prevents the precise quantification of risks and benefits that might help to make an informed decision about trial of labor compared with elective repeat cesarean delivery. The panel was mindful of these clinical and ethical uncertainties in making the following conclusions and recommendations.

One of the panel's major goals is to support pregnant women with one prior transverse uterine incision to make informed decisions about trial of labor compared with elective repeat cesarean delivery. The panel recommends that clinicians and other maternity care providers use the responses to the six questions, especially questions 3 and 4, to incorporate an evidence-based approach into the decisionmaking process. Information, including risk assessment, should be shared with the woman at a level and pace that she can understand. When trial of labor and elective repeat cesarean delivery are medically equivalent options, a shared decisionmaking process should be adopted and, whenever possible, the woman's preference should be honored.

The panel is concerned about the barriers that women face in gaining access to clinicians and facilities that are able and willing to offer trial of labor. Given the low level of evidence for the requirement for "immediately available" surgical and anesthesia personnel in current guidelines, the panel recommends that the American College of Obstetricians and Gynecologists and the American Society of Anesthesiologists reassess this requirement with specific reference to other obstetric complications of comparable risk, risk stratification, and in light of limited physician and nursing resources. Healthcare organizations, physicians, and other clinicians should consider making public their trial of labor policies and VBAC rates, as well as their plans for responding to obstetric emergencies. The panel recommends that hospitals, maternity care providers, healthcare and professional liability insurers, consumers, and policymakers collaborate on the development of integrated services that could mitigate or even eliminate current barriers to trial of labor.

The panel is concerned that medical-legal considerations add to, and in many instances exacerbate, these barriers to trial of labor. Policymakers, providers, and other stakeholders must collaborate in developing and implementing appropriate strategies to mitigate the chilling effect the medical-legal environment has on access to care.

High-quality research is needed in many areas. The panel has identified areas that need attention in response to question 6. Research in these areas should be given appropriate priority and should be adequately funded— especially studies that would help to characterize more precisely the short-term and long-term maternal, fetal, and neonatal outcomes of trial of labor and elective repeat cesarean delivery.

Introduction

Vaginal birth after cesarean (VBAC) describes vaginal delivery by a woman who has had a previous cesarean delivery. For most of the 20th century, once a woman had undergone a cesarean delivery, clinicians believed that her future pregnancies required cesarean delivery. Studies from the 1960s suggested that this practice may not always be necessary. In 1980, a National Institutes of Health (NIH) Consensus Development Conference Panel questioned the necessity of routine repeat cesarean deliveries and outlined situations in which VBAC could be considered. The option for a woman with a previous cesarean delivery to have a trial of labor was offered and exercised more often in the 1980s through 1996. Since 1996, however, the number of VBACs has declined, contributing to the overall increase in cesarean delivery (Figure 1). Although we recognize that primary cesarean deliveries are the driving force behind the total cesarean delivery rates, the focus of this report is on trial of labor and *repeat* cesarean deliveries.

Figure 1. Rates of Total Cesarean Deliveries, Primary Cesarean Deliveries, and VBAC, 1989–2007

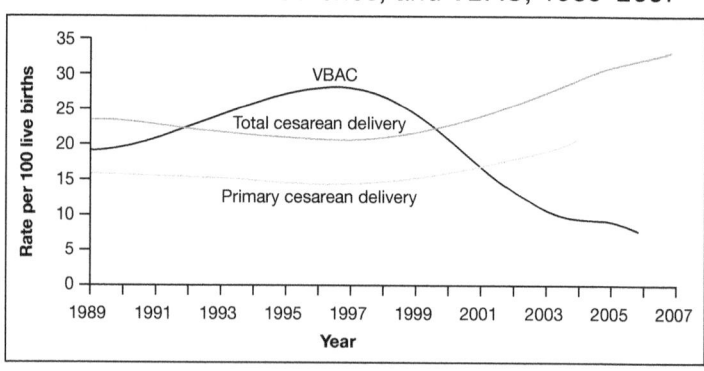

Data from the National Center for Health Statistics.

A number of medical and nonmedical factors have contributed to this decline in the VBAC rate since the mid-1990s, although many of these factors are not well understood. A significant medical factor that is frequently cited as a reason to avoid trial of labor is concern about the possibility of uterine rupture—because an unsuccessful trial of labor, in which a woman undergoes a repeat cesarean delivery instead of a vaginal delivery, has a a higher rate of complications compared to VBAC or elective repeat cesarean delivery. Nonmedical factors include, among other things, restrictions on access to a trial of labor and the effect of the current medical-legal climate on relevant practice patterns. To advance understanding of these important issues, the *Eunice Kennedy Shriver* National Institute of Child Health and Human Development and the Office of Medical Applications of Research of NIH convened a Consensus Development Conference on March 8–10, 2010. The conference was grounded in the view that a thorough evaluation of the relevant research would help pregnant women and their maternity care providers when making decisions about the mode of delivery after a previous cesarean delivery. Improved understanding of the clinical risks and benefits and how they interact with nonmedical factors also may have important implications for informed decisionmaking and health services planning.

The following key questions were addressed by the Consensus Development Conference:

1. What are the rates and patterns of utilization of trial of labor after prior cesarean delivery, vaginal birth after cesarean delivery, and repeat cesarean delivery in the United States?

2. Among women who attempt a trial of labor after prior cesarean delivery, what is the vaginal delivery rate and the factors that influence it?

3. What are the short- and long-term benefits and harms to the mother of attempting trial of labor after prior cesarean versus elective repeat cesarean delivery, and what factors influence benefits and harms?

4. What are the short- and long-term benefits and harms to the baby of maternal attempt at trial of labor after prior cesarean versus elective repeat cesarean delivery, and what factors influence benefits and harms?

5. What are the nonmedical factors that influence the patterns and utilization of trial of labor after prior cesarean delivery?

6. What are the critical gaps in the evidence for decisionmaking, and what are the priority investigations needed to address these gaps?

Invited experts presented information pertinent to the posed questions and a systematic literature review prepared under contract with AHRQ, available at **http://www.ahrq.gov/clinic/tp/vbacuptp.htm**, was summarized. Conference attendees asked questions and provided comments. After weighing the scientific evidence, an unbiased, independent panel prepared this consensus statement.

Pregnant women, clinicians, and investigators use terms in conflicting and confusing ways. For consistency throughout this document, the following definitions are provided:

- Trial of labor: A planned attempt to labor by a woman who has had a previous cesarean delivery, also known as trial of labor after cesarean.

- Vaginal birth after cesarean delivery (VBAC): Vaginal delivery after a trial of labor; that is, a successful trial of labor.

- Unsuccessful trial of labor: Delivery by cesarean delivery in a woman who has had a trial of labor; sometimes referred to as a "failed" trial of labor.

- Elective repeat cesarean delivery: Planned cesarean delivery by a woman who has had one or more prior cesarean deliveries. The delivery may or may not be scheduled.

Data in this statement are presented using trial of labor as the reference group compared to elective repeat cesarean delivery. We emphasize that some data refer to women with trial of labor irrespective of mode of delivery (VBAC or unsuccessful trial of labor), and some comparisons refer to women who had VBAC compared to those who had repeat cesarean delivery (unsuccessful trial of labor and elective repeat cesarean delivery). These distinctions are made when possible. Also, the evidence is summarized by presenting outcomes with high or moderate grade of evidence first, followed by low grade, then absent data.[1] We intentionally identify outcomes without supporting data to stimulate further research and highlight the variety of important issues that may not be well studied, but that women and their maternity care providers face when deciding on trial of labor compared with elective repeat cesarean delivery.

---

[1] The strength of evidence was graded. High grade of evidence (future research unlikely to change estimate) is defined as having multiple high-quality studies in applicable patients with consistent results. Moderate grade of evidence (future research may change estimate) is defined as having a moderate confidence in studies such that additional studies may change the estimate. Low grade of evidence (research likely to change effect size or direction) is defined as having a low number of studies or serious flaws in study design or applicability of subgroups. Insufficient evidence indicates either no evidence or inability to estimate the effect. (Definitions from the U.S. Preventive Services Task Force.)

1. What Are the Rates and Patterns of Utilization of Trial of Labor After Prior Cesarean, Vaginal Birth After Cesarean, and Repeat Cesarean Delivery in the United States?

The overall cesarean delivery rate is the sum of primary and repeat cesarean deliveries per 100 live births. Following a decline between 1990 and 1996, cesarean delivery rates in the United States rose markedly from 21 percent in 1996 to 32 percent in 2007 (see Figure 1). Both the primary and repeat cesarean birth rates have risen. Among women with a prior cesarean delivery, VBAC rates vary by racial/ethnic status, medical condition, region of the country, type and location of hospital, and may vary by type of provider. For Medicaid patients, VBAC rates are higher for women enrolled in health maintenance organizations or who deliver at public (not private) hospitals. Various surveys have revealed that since 1996, approximately one-third of hospitals and one-half of physicians no longer offer trial of labor. A survey of American College of Obstetricians and Gynecologists Fellows showed that, between 2003 and 2006, 26 percent stopped offering a trial of labor for women with a history of cesarean deliveries regardless of prior vaginal delivery experience.

A woman is at low risk for pregnancy complications if she has completed 37 weeks of gestation with one fetus whose head is in the vertex position in the womb and has no obstetric or medical complications. Among low-risk women, the repeat cesarean delivery rate had increased to 89 percent by 2003. Since 2003, U.S. Standard Birth Certificates have included information on VBAC and trial of labor. Among the 19 states that had adopted the standard certificate, approximately 92 percent of all women who had a previous cesarean had a repeat cesarean for their next delivery in 2006. A sharp rise in repeat cesareans was observed at all maternal ages and for all racial/ethnic groups.

Given these trends, VBAC is an important issue to explore. Although the number of women and their maternity care providers faced with the question of whether to attempt trial of labor has markedly increased, there has been a concurrent, dramatic drop in VBAC. Yet cesarean and VBAC rates are identified as quality indicators for maternal health by policymakers, insurance providers, and healthcare quality monitoring groups. Success of trial of labor is consistently high, ranging from 60 to 80 percent, whereas the risk of uterine rupture is low, at less than 1 percent. Regardless, one reason given for reduced VBAC is concern about uterine rupture during trial of labor.

Little is known about population-based rates and patterns of utilization of trial of labor after previous cesarean deliveries. A potential source of information about this issue is the Pregnancy Risk Assessment Monitoring System (PRAMS), an ongoing surveillance program conducted by the Centers for Disease Control and Prevention and state health departments. PRAMS is a population-based survey of a sample of women who have recently delivered. Each year, a relatively small sample of postpartum women is selected in each state (n=1,300 to n=3,400). In addition to a core questionnaire, participating states may choose to supplement from a set of standard questions or derive questions of their own.

New Jersey represents a good example of the use of birth data. New Jersey tracked trial of labor and repeat cesareans from 1997 to 2008 using electronic birth systems. Over this time period, there has been an increase in repeat cesarean deliveries from less than 50 percent to nearly 85 percent. There was very little difference in this rate between women with or without private insurance or by maternal risk status. Between 2003 and 2005, 79 percent of low-risk women in New Jersey underwent repeat cesarean delivery without a trial of labor. Since 2009, New Jersey has been utilizing PRAMS to learn more about mothers' and providers' predelivery intentions for VBAC and informed consent for type of delivery.

In summary, in states where data are collected, VBAC has dropped dramatically since 1996. Although the data among racial/ethnic groups vary, repeat cesarean deliveries without trial of labor have increased in all these groups. Rates of repeat cesarean continue to increase even among women who are low risk.

2. Among Women Who Attempt a Trial of Labor After Prior Cesarean, What Is the Vaginal Delivery Rate and the Factors That Influence It?

Although the trial of labor rate has declined dramatically over the past several decades, the vaginal delivery rate after trial of labor has remained constant at approximately 74 percent. The reported rates are highly variable, the overall strength of the body of evidence is moderate, and most studies use data from large tertiary care and training centers. In addition, many studies are observational and do not adequately address issues of selection bias. Confounding and inadequate measurement of variables are a concern. Taken together, these methodological and statistical issues limit the strength of the information available.

Many demographic and obstetric factors are associated with the likelihood of VBAC. Race and ethnicity are the strongest demographic predictors of vaginal delivery after trial of labor. Hispanic and African American women have lower rates of VBAC than non-Hispanic white women. Increasing maternal age, single marital status, and less than 12 years of education also have been associated with lower rates of VBAC. Women who deliver at rural and private hospitals and the presence of maternal disease (e.g., hypertension, diabetes, asthma, seizures, renal disease, thyroid disease, heart disease) may also be associated with a decreased likelihood of VBAC. Greater maternal height and body mass index below 30 kg/m2 are associated with an increased likelihood of VBAC.

A prior history of vaginal delivery, either before or after a prior cesarean delivery, is consistently associated with an increased likelihood of VBAC. For example, in one retrospective cohort study, the vaginal birth rate after trial of labor was 63 percent in women with no prior vaginal delivery, 83 percent in women with a prior vaginal delivery before cesarean delivery, and 94 percent in women with a prior VBAC. The rate of VBAC increases with each prior VBAC. Nonrecurring indications for cesarean delivery are also associated with a higher rate of VBAC. For example, compared to arrest of labor, prior cesarean delivery for malpresentation is associated with a higher rate of VBAC. Women who previously delivered babies weighing less than 4,000 grams are more likely to have a VBAC than are those who delivered heavier babies.

Current pregnancy factors also are associated with vaginal delivery after trial of labor, including labor characteristics and infant factors. Gestational age greater than 40 weeks, labor augmentation, and labor induction are associated with a decreased rate of VBAC. The most consistent infant factor associated with an increased likelihood of VBAC is birth weight less than 4,000 grams. Lower gestational age at delivery is associated with increased VBAC rates when compared to term gestational age at delivery. Labor factors associated with a higher VBAC rate include greater cervical dilation at admission or at rupture of membranes. The likelihood of VBAC increases if cervical effacement reaches 75 to 90 percent. Vertex position, fetal head engagement or a lower station, and higher Bishop score (a scoring system used to estimate the success of induction of labor) also increase the likelihood of VBAC. Data regarding epidural analgesia and VBAC are inconsistent.

A major area of interest is whether antepartum or intrapartum management strategies—for example, methods of labor induction—influence the rate of VBAC. The overall estimated rate of vaginal birth after any method of labor induction is 63 percent. Studies demonstrate that the rate of VBAC ranges from 54 percent for induction of labor with mechanical (transcervical balloon catheter) to 69 percent for induction with pharmacologic methods. The majority of studies were conducted in large, tertiary care settings, and many studies were conducted outside the United States. Results were not stratified by age, race, ethnicity, or baseline risk. Rigorous studies have not compared VBAC rates with different induction methods.

Several screening tools have been proposed for predicting VBAC. These tools take into account factors such as maternal age, body mass index, prior vaginal delivery, prior cesarean indication, cervical dilation, and effacement at admission. The models have reasonable ability to predict the likelihood of a successful trial of labor at the population level but are not accurate in predicting the risk of a uterine rupture or unsuccessful trial of labor. Studies have not verified the utility of these screening tools for predicting outcomes for individual women.

3. What Are the Short- and Long-Term Benefits and Harms to the Mother of Attempting Trial of Labor After Prior Cesarean Versus Elective Repeat Cesarean Delivery, and What Factors Influence Benefits and Harms?

Overall, pregnancy and birth have inherent risks and benefits. There is controversy regarding the risks and benefits of cesarean delivery, and little high-quality evidence is available about benefits and harms of trial of labor and elective repeat cesarean delivery specifically. A previous NIH State-of-the-Science Conference (*http://consensus.nih.gov/2006/cesarean.htm*) partially addressed the global issues related to benefits and harms of cesarean compared to vaginal delivery, which is out of the scope of this review. Ideally, for the purposes of counseling women with a prior cesarean delivery about their options for mode of delivery, data from women who gave birth at term should be used. Unfortunately, insufficient data are available about women at term only; thus, this review includes data on outcomes related to trial of labor compared with elective repeat cesarean delivery for all women who give birth at all gestational ages. When data are available for term gestations only, these data are presented separately.

Limitations to these findings include differing definitions for the outcomes, heterogeneity among studies, and variation in study designs. Mortality and morbidity of trial of labor and elective repeat cesarean delivery are likely to be underestimated due to reporting bias and the potential for missing complications that occur after discharge. The major outcomes reflecting benefits and harms of trial of labor are presented in **bold font** and in descending order of grade of evidence within this section. However, the factors influencing these outcomes do not always hold the same level of evidence, which is highlighted in each section below.

For women with a prior cesarean delivery, there are three possible outcomes: a VBAC (i.e., a successful trial of labor), an unsuccessful trial of labor resulting in cesarean delivery, or an elective repeat cesarean delivery. In general, the overall *benefits* of trial of labor are directly related to having a VBAC, because these women typically have the lowest morbidity. Similarly, the *harms* of trial of labor are associated with an unsuccessful trial of labor resulting in cesarean delivery, because these deliveries have the highest morbidity. Although there is merit in studying each of these three groups separately, the data comparing trial of labor to elective repeat cesarean delivery that were reviewed for this conference typically combined VBAC and unsuccessful trial of labor ending in cesarean delivery. Consequently, the health outcomes reported below for women who have an unsuccessful trial of labor and subsequently undergo repeat cesarean delivery are counted in the overall trial of labor cohort(s). This approach best reflects the knowledge that is available to women who have had a previous cesarean delivery at the time they are deciding on the subsequent mode of delivery for a current pregnancy.

SHORT-TERM BENEFITS FOR TRIAL OF LABOR

High Grade of Evidence

Maternal mortality is low, but it may be increasing in the United States. Women who have a trial of labor, regardless of ultimate mode of delivery, are at decreased risk of maternal mortality compared to elective repeat cesarean delivery. Although there is some heterogeneity among studies reporting death in term only compared to any gestational age, overall estimates of maternal death number 3.8 per 100,000 for women who undergo a trial of labor compared with 13.4 per 100,000 live births for elective repeat cesarean delivery (Table 1). At term, these numbers decrease to 1.9 (trial of labor) compared with 9.6 (elective repeat cesarean delivery) maternal deaths per 100,000 live births. Studies of factors affecting maternal mortality with trial of labor and elective repeat cesarean delivery are of low-grade evidence; however, they imply lower mortality for trial of labor in high-volume hospitals (more than 500 deliveries per year). Table 1 puts into perspective the death rates of mothers in the population of women with prior cesarean, relative to other common causes of death in the general population.

Table 1. Mortality Rates

	Overall	Trial of Labor Prior Cesarean Delivery	Elective Repeat Cesarean Prior Cesarean Delivery
All-cause mortality in women by age (per 100,000 total U.S. population)*			
15–24 years	42		
25–34 years	64		
35–44 years	136		
Motor vehicle-related mortality (per 100,000 total U.S. population)(Men and women, 25–44 years)*	16		
Maternal mortality (pregnancy to delivery, all ages, per 100,000 live births)*	13		
Maternal mortality in women with prior cesarean, all ages, at delivery, per 100,000 live births†		4	13

* U.S. 2007 National Center for Health Statistics data.
†Data from supporting systematic evidence review.

The overall risk of **hysterectomy** is statistically similar for trial of labor compared with elective repeat cesarean delivery (157 versus 280 per 100,000, respectively) and may be less in women at term. Limited evidence suggests that the risk of hysterectomy increases with induction of labor, high-risk pregnancy, and increasing number of cesarean deliveries (420 for one prior cesarean delivery, 900 for two prior cesarean deliveries, 2,410 for three prior cesarean deliveries, 3,490 for four prior cesarean deliveries, and 8,990 for five or more prior cesarean deliveries per 100,000). The risk of **blood transfusion** is not significantly different for trial of labor or elective repeat cesarean delivery

(900 versus 1,200 per 100,000, respectively). Factors that increase this risk include induction of labor with no prior vaginal delivery, high-risk pregnancy, and an increased number of prior cesarean deliveries.

There is shorter **hospitalization** overall for trial of labor compared to elective repeat cesarean delivery. This benefit does not pertain to morbidly obese women. A single study suggests lower rates of **deep venous thrombosis (DVT)** in women undergoing trial of labor compared with elective repeat cesarean delivery (40 versus 100 per 100,000, respectively).

A woman's perceptions of her birth experience, initial parent-infant interactions, and ability to perform activities of daily living or initiate breastfeeding may differ by mode of delivery. There are insufficient comparative studies in women with a prior cesarean delivery to address these issues.

None

Uterine rupture is defined as an anatomic separation of the uterine muscle with or without symptoms. Although uncommon, this event can be catastrophic and remains the most dreaded short-term complication of trial of labor. The concern for uterine rupture is an important factor affecting counseling regarding risks and benefits of trial of labor. There is a clear increased risk of uterine rupture in women who have a trial of labor compared to elective repeat cesarean delivery. The presence of a uterine rupture has numerous adverse consequences for both mother and baby.

Incidence of Uterine Rupture

Considering all gestational ages, uterine rupture occurs in approximately 325 per 100,000 women undergoing trial of labor. The risk of uterine rupture for women who undergo trial of labor at term is 778 per 100,000. The risk of uterine rupture for women who undergo elective repeat cesarean delivery is 26 per 100,000 when all gestational ages are evaluated and 22 per 100,000 for women who are at term at the time they give birth. Unfortunately, there is no reliable way to predict who will have a uterine rupture.

Factors That Increase the Risk of Uterine Rupture

The following discussion of factors that affect the risk of uterine rupture is based on **low-grade evidence**.

Women with **classical and low vertical uterine scars** have an increased risk of rupture when compared to women who had a low transverse uterine incision at the time of cesarean delivery. **Induction of labor** has been associated with uterine rupture. However, due to variation among studies with respect to indications for delivery, induction protocol, agent and dose, and subsequent use of oxytocin, it is difficult to identify an absolute risk of uterine rupture associated with induction. The risk of rupture in women at term who have their labor induced is higher (1,500 per 100,000) than the risk of rupture if labor starts spontaneously (800 per 100,000). The risk of rupture may be increased in women who are induced at more than 40 weeks (3,200 per 100,000 at more than 40 weeks versus 1,500 per 100,000 at 37 to 40 weeks). There does not appear to be an increased risk of rupture with oxytocin augmentation of spontaneous labor.

A recently published meta-analysis revealed that an **increase in the number of prior cesarean deliveries** may increase the risks of uterine rupture; two or more previous cesarean deliveries were associated with higher rupture rates (1,590 per 100,000) than one prior cesarean delivery (560 per 100,000). **Other factors** that may increase the risk of uterine rupture include unfavorable cervical status at the time of admission, obesity, inter-pregnancy interval of 18 months or less, single-layer closure for the initial cesarean delivery, an infant weighing more than 4,000 grams, and giving birth in a low-volume hospital. Insufficient data are available to quantify the specific effects of these factors.

Factors That Decrease the Risk of Uterine Rupture

A **prior vaginal birth** (before or after the previous cesarean delivery) decreases the risk of uterine rupture to approximately 600 per 100,000.

Consequences of Uterine Rupture

There have been no reported maternal deaths due to uterine rupture. Overall, 14 to 33 percent of women will need a hysterectomy when the uterus ruptures. Approximately 6 percent of uterine ruptures will result in perinatal death. This is an overall risk of intrapartum fetal death of 20 per 100,000 women undergoing trial of labor. For term pregnancies, the reported risk of fetal death with uterine rupture is less than 3 percent. Although the risk is similarly low, there is insufficient evidence to quantify the neonatal morbidity directly related to uterine rupture.

Insufficient Evidence for Short-Term Harm

Reported rates of **infection** vary widely depending on the definitions used. Overall, the rates of infection are low (below 3 percent or less than 3,000 per 100,000) with increased trends toward higher infection rates with trial of labor. Morbid obesity, unsuccessful trial of labor, and increased number of cesarean deliveries increase infection rates. Evidence is sparse for rates of short-term **surgical injury**. There do not appear to be differences between trial of labor and elective repeat cesarean delivery, but surgical injury increases with unsuccessful trial of labor, vertical abdominal incision (as opposed to Pfannenstiel incision), and increasing number of cesarean deliveries.

LONG-TERM BENEFITS OF TRIAL OF LABOR

High Grade of Evidence

None

Moderate Grade of Evidence

There is an association between cesarean delivery and **abnormal placental position and growth** in subsequent pregnancies and the risk of having abnormal placental position and growth increases with increasing number of cesarean deliveries. Although most women in the United States have two or fewer births, the chance of having abnormal placental position or growth in subsequent pregnancy are of great concern for the 28 percent of women who have more than two births. An important aspect in counseling women about trial of labor compared with elective repeat cesarean delivery should therefore include the woman's plans for future fertility.

For the purposes of comparing outcomes between trial of labor and elective repeat cesarean delivery, it is recognized that all these women have had at least one cesarean delivery, and are at baseline higher risk for abnormal placental position and growth compared to women who have not had a cesarean delivery. Overall, the major benefit of trial of labor is the 74 percent likelihood of VBAC and avoidance of multiple cesarean deliveries. However, women who have an unsuccessful trial of labor and repeat cesarean delivery do not realize the benefit of decreased risk for abnormal placental position or growth in subsequent pregnancies. The following health outcomes occur **less frequently** in women who have a VBAC (i.e., a successful trial of labor) and are of most concern for women who have more than two births.

The incidence of **placenta previa** (placenta covering the cervix) significantly increases in women with each additional cesarean delivery, occurring in 900 per 100,000 women who have one prior cesarean delivery, 1,700 per 100,000 women who have two prior cesarean deliveries, and 3,000 per 100,000 in women who have three or more cesarean deliveries. As the number of cesarean deliveries increase, major morbidity, including placenta accreta and hysterectomy, also increase when a pleacenta previa is present.

Even in the absence of placenta previa, the incidence of **placenta accreta, increta, and percreta** (growth of the placenta into or through the uterine muscle) increases with the number of cesarean deliveries. This has a profound effect on the woman's future reproductive capability. The baseline risk of placenta accreta in a woman with one prior cesarean delivery is 319 per 100,000; this increases to 570 per 100,000 for two prior cesarean deliveries, and approximately 2,400 per 100,000 for three or more cesarean deliveries. No factors have been identified to decrease this risk. There does not appear to be an increased incidence of **placental abruption** (i.e., premature separation of the normally implanted placenta from the uterus) with increasing number of cesarean deliveries, although the risk is increased when women who have one prior cesarean delivery are compared to women who have not had a cesarean delivery.

Low Grade of Evidence

None

Although cesarean delivery has been implicated in **other conditions** such as chronic pain, ectopic pregnancy, stillbirth, and infertility, there are no studies examining these conditions in women with prior cesarean delivery with respect to trial of labor compared with elective repeat cesarean delivery. With respect to **complications related to subsequent surgery**, no studies have specifically compared trial of labor with elective repeat cesarean delivery. However, it is generally recognized that an increasing number of abdominal surgeries is associated with the following complications: clinically significant adhesions, perioperative complications at time of subsequent repeat cesarean delivery, bowel and ureteral injuries, and perioperative complications at time of non-pregnancy-related hysterectomy.

LONG-TERM HARMS OF TRIAL OF LABOR

High or Moderate Grades of Evidence

None

Low Grade of Evidence

None

Insufficient Evidence for Long-Term Harm

No studies on long-term **pelvic floor function** have compared women who have a trial of labor with women who have an elective repeat cesarean delivery. Although women who experience a vaginal delivery may have increased risks of pelvic floor disorders, such as stress incontinence or pelvic organ prolapse, compared to women who have a cesarean delivery, the labor progress and timing of the original cesarean delivery influence these risks. As such, elective repeat cesarean delivery for the prevention of pelvic floor disorders should not be considered protective against stress incontinence and prolapse.

4. What Are the Short- and Long-Term Benefits and Harms to the Baby of Maternal Attempt at Trial of Labor After Prior Cesarean Versus Elective Repeat Cesarean Delivery, and What Factors Influence Benefits and Harms?

The discussion between women and their maternity care providers about whether to proceed with elective repeat cesarean delivery or trial of labor following prior cesarean delivery must assess potential benefits and harms for both mother and fetus. In contrast to the data on maternal outcomes, there is little or no evidence on short- or long-term neonatal outcomes after trial of labor compared to elective repeat cesarean delivery. Much of the evidence is of low quality, characterized by inconsistencies in outcomes across studies and differences in outcome definitions, and variations in study design. However, there are extensive data documenting differences in neonatal outcomes following vaginal delivery compared to cesarean delivery in general. Overall, following cesarean delivery, infants have increased rates of short-term respiratory sequelae, interference with initial mother-infant contact, and delayed breastfeeding initiation compared to infants born vaginally. Long-term consequences may include asthma. However, there are little data on these outcomes when trial of labor and elective repeat cesarean delivery are compared in women who had a prior cesarean delivery. Furthermore, there are essentially no data on factors contributing to neonatal benefits and harms. The major outcomes reflecting benefits and harms of trial of labor compared to elective repeat cesarean delivery are presented in **bold font** and in descending order of grade of evidence within this section.

SHORT-TERM OUTCOMES

High Grade of Evidence

None

Studies of **perinatal mortality** (death between 20 weeks of gestation and 28 days of life) are of moderate quality and show that the perinatal mortality rate is increased for trial of labor at 130 per 100,000 compared to elective repeat cesarean delivery at 50 per 100,000. Although this difference is statistically significant, the magnitude of the difference between the two groups is small and comparable to the perinatal mortality rate observed among laboring nulliparous women. The **neonatal mortality rate** (death in the first 28 days of life) is 110 per 100,000 for trial of labor compared to 50 per 100,000 for elective repeat cesarean delivery (Table 2). Table 2 puts into perspective the death rates of babies in the population of women with prior cesarean delivery, relative to other causes of death.

Table 2. Mortality Rates per 100,000 Infants

	Overall	Trial of Labor Prior Cesarean Delivery	Elective Repeat Cesarean Delivery Prior Cesarean Delivery
All-cause mortality <1 year*	677		
Sudden infant death syndrome (SIDS)*	49		
Perinatal mortality from >20 weeks' gestation to <28 days postbirth*	1,073		
Perinatal mortality in women with prior cesarean, at delivery†		130	50

* U.S. 2007 National Center for Health Statistics data.
†Data from supporting systematic evidence review.

Studies of **fetal mortality** (deaths *in utero* at 20 weeks of gestation or greater) are of low quality and suggest a higher death rate in trial of labor at 50 to 130 per 100,000 compared to elective repeat cesarean delivery at 0 to 40 per 100,000. Elective repeat cesarean delivery may have contributed to the reduction of stillbirths that occur in the late third trimester and the decline in perinatal mortality observed over the last two decades, because elective repeat cesarean delivery is rarely performed after 40 weeks, whereas women who undergo trial of labor may have longer gestations.

Hypoxic ischemic encephalopathy in term infants has an incidence of 100 per 100,000 live births. That said, it is considered one of the most catastrophic outcomes and is one contributor to long-term neurological impairment in infants. Such neurological damage is one of the most serious adverse consequences of uterine rupture and a major reason why women and clinicians are concerned about electing trial of labor. The systematic evidence review reported insufficient data on the incidence of hypoxic ischemic encephalopathy between infants born following trial of labor compared with elective repeat cesarean delivery. However, a recent observational study of more than 33,000 women found a significantly higher incidence of hypoxic ischemic encephalopathy in trial of labor compared with elective repeat cesarean delivery (12 cases versus 0 cases, respectively, or 46 per 100,000 for trial of labor compared with 0 per 100,000 for elective repeat cesarean delivery). Unfortunately, the studies on this important outcome are limited by inconsistency in study methodology.

Insufficient Evidence

Infants born by elective repeat cesarean delivery may have higher rates of **respiratory sequelae**, including respiratory distress syndrome, transient tachypnea of the newborn, and need for oxygen and ventilator support when compared to infants born by VBAC. There is a lack of data to determine whether substantial differences in respiratory outcomes occur in infants born via elective repeat cesarean delivery compared with infants born after trial of labor to women who had a prior cesarean.

Studies of **sepsis** were of low quality. No meaningful conclusions could be drawn.

Infants born by elective repeat cesarean delivery are at increased risk for **birth trauma** such as fetal lacerations. Studies of brachial plexus injury (upper extremity nerve injury) show an incidence of 180 per 100,000 in infants born by VBAC compared to 30 per 100,000 among infants born by elective repeat cesarean delivery. However, there does not appear to be a substantial difference in persistent neurological impairment after brachial plexus injury between trial of labor and elective repeat cesarean delivery.

No comparative data exist on **breastfeeding** practices among women who had a prior cesarean delivery who undergo trial of labor compared with elective repeat cesarean delivery.

Comparative data regarding factors affecting **mother-infant bonding**, including the long-term well-being of the infant and early mother-infant contact, are lacking for women undergoing trial of labor or elective repeat cesarean delivery.

5. What Are the Nonmedical Factors That Influence the Patterns and Utilization of Trial of Labor After Prior Cesarean?

We considered the influence of the following nonmedical factors on practice and utilization patterns related to trial of labor:

- Professional association practice guidelines

- Professional liability concerns among physicians and hospitals

- The nature and extent of informed decisionmaking

- Provider and birth-setting issues

- Health insurance status and insurance reimbursement

- Patient and provider preferences.

The literature syntheses that informed this consensus conference did not include these issues as part of the evidence-based systematic review. Even so, we have concluded that they are important influences on access to trial of labor. We have also concluded that data are not available to judge the *relative* impact of these various factors or how they interact.

Professional Association Practice Guidelines

In 1999, the American College of Obstetricians and Gynecologists (the College) released a practice guideline changing its earlier recommendation of "encouraging" VBAC to a recommendation that women should be "offered" trial of labor if there are no contraindications. The guideline also stated that trial of labor should be performed only in institutions equipped to respond to obstetric emergencies and in settings where physicians capable of performing a cesarean delivery are "immediately available" to provide emergency care. According to the College, evidence to support this guideline was rated as Level C (based on consensus and expert opinion). Not all institutions were able to comply with this new standard, which in turn led some to cease offering trial of labor and therefore VBAC altogether.

Two recent surveys of hospital administrators found that 30 percent of hospitals stopped providing trial of labor services because they could not provide immediate surgical and anesthesia services. Some have referred to these policies as "VBAC bans." Of the hospitals that still offer trial of labor, more than half had to change their policies to comply with the 1999 College recommendation.

A joint statement by the American College of Obstetricians and Gynecologists and the American Society of

Anesthesiologists in 2008 also called for the "immediate availability of appropriate facilities and personnel, including obstetric anesthesia, nursing personnel, and a physician capable of monitoring labor and performing cesarean delivery, including an emergency cesarean delivery, in cases of vaginal birth after cesarean delivery."

Even so, experts in tracking anesthesia staff resources have found that there are too few anesthesia providers to ensure "immediate" anesthesia availability for all hospitals providing childbirth services. Moreover, they predict that these shortages will worsen in the future.

Professional Liability Concerns Among Physicians and Hospitals

Concerns over liability risk have a major impact on the willingness of physicians and healthcare institutions to offer trial of labor. These concerns derive from the perception that catastrophic events associated with trial of labor could lead to compensable claims with large verdicts or settlements for fetal/maternal injury— regardless of the adequacy of informed consent. Clearly, these medical malpractice issues affect practice patterns among healthcare providers and they played a role in the genesis of the College's 1999 "immediately available" guideline.

Members of the American College of Obstetricians and Gynecologists confirm that concern over liability is a main reason they stopped offering trial of labor. A 2009 College survey revealed that 30 percent of obstetricians stopped offering trial of labor or performing VBACs because of the risk or fear of professional liability claims or litigation. This is further compounded by 29 percent acknowledging having increased their number of cesarean deliveries and 8 percent having stopped practicing obstetrics altogether. In a recent study of College Fellows, risk of liability was among the primary reasons cited for performing a cesarean delivery.

In addition, studies have attempted to model the impact of tort reform on primary and repeat cesarean delivery rates and have shown that modest improvements in the medical-legal climate may result in increases in VBAC and reductions in cesarean deliveries. These analyses suggest that both caps on noneconomic damages and reductions in physician malpractice premiums would result in fewer cesarean deliveries.

The Nature and Extent of Informed Decisionmaking

It is important that women understand the spectrum of risks and benefits of trial of labor and elective repeat cesarean delivery, given the evidence that providing such information has a significant impact on a woman's ability to make an informed choice about whether or not trial of labor is a reasonable option for her. Several studies suggest that *how* risk is presented and communicated by providers has a powerful effect on women's decisions. Along these same lines, the 1999 College guideline urged, "After thorough counseling that weighs the individual benefits and risks of VBAC, the ultimate decision to attempt this procedure or undergo a repeat caesarean delivery should be made by the woman and her physician." Presentations at the conference suggested that this important recommended practice is not uniformly followed, but there are no strong data documenting the extent of this shortcoming.

Patterns and use of trial of labor also may reflect women's varying levels of knowledge and appreciation about the benefits and risks of the particular delivery options available. More generally, there is limited public understanding of the baseline risks of pregnancy and childbirth in general.

A variety of decision aids are available to help women understand the risks, benefits, and implications of trial of labor compared with elective repeat cesarean delivery. A few well-designed studies suggest that certain tools can increase women's knowledge, reduce their anxiety, and help them in their decisionmaking process.

Provider and Birth-Setting Issues

No strong comparative data are available to assess the relative impact of types of maternity care providers (obstetrician-gynecologists, family practice physicians, midwives) on patterns and utilization of trial of labor after controlling for selection bias and patient mix.

Some evidence shows that younger obstetric providers are less willing and interested in offering trial of labor. This may reflect the fact that their training occurred at a time when trial of labor was steadily decreasing.

Women give birth in a variety of settings in and out of hospitals, including tertiary care centers, community hospitals, freestanding birth centers, and at home. Most data on maternal and neonatal outcomes are collected in tertiary care settings, which means that there is little data that assesses these outcomes across numerous settings. However, there is a positive association between settings with a high volume of deliveries and better outcomes, especially lower rates of neonatal mortality in premature infants.

Health Insurance and Reimbursement

Current data do not allow clear conclusions to be made about the effect a woman's health insurance status has on her access to trial of labor. It also is not clear whether overall reimbursement levels for VBAC compared with elective repeat cesarean delivery have a major influence on either hospital or physician practice patterns.

Patient and Provider Preferences

As a general matter, women report that their preferences regarding delivery options are influenced by their maternity care providers' recommendations and concerns about safety, including a desire for a healthy baby and fear of a bad outcome.

Factors linked to women's preference for pursuing trial of labor include self-reported desire for their partners' involvement, a sense that labor and vaginal delivery can be deeply empowering, maternal-infant bonding, greater ease in breastfeeding, and the expectation of an easier recovery. Conversely, a desire for sterilization at time of delivery, scheduling convenience, a preference for elective repeat cesarean delivery over emergency cesarean delivery or operative vaginal delivery, the desire to avoid labor pain, and fear of an unsuccessful trial of labor have been identified as reasons for preferring a scheduled repeat cesarean delivery. The role of other factors in women's preferences—including how the risk of uterine rupture is viewed, sociodemographic status, social norms, values, and beliefs—are less well understood.

With regard to health care provider preferences, few data exist to assess how obstetric providers view offering both options (trial of labor and elective repeat cesarean delivery) to their patients (holding other factors constant such as liability concerns or past experience) and the conditions under which they would feel comfortable engaging their patients in a thoughtful process of shared decisionmaking.

6. What Are the Critical Gaps in the Evidence for Decisionmaking, and What Are the Priority Investigations Needed to Address These Gaps?

Critical gap 1: There is a need for uniform and simple-to-use definitions that would be common to all data collection. We recommend a standardized and systematic use of definitions for short-term and long-term maternal and neonatal outcomes.

Critical gap 2: There appear to be persistent racial/ethnic, geographic, and socioeconomic differences in the rate of trial of labor and VBAC compared with elective repeat cesarean delivery. We recommend investigation to understand the reasons for these differences.

Critical gap 3: The factors that affect the course of labor and its clinical management are incompletely understood. We recommend well-designed clinical studies on practice variation, provider type and setting, and intrapartum management including induction methods. Methodologies should be developed that address the challenges of conducting studies based on plans for delivery, which can change during the course of pregnancy.

Critical gap 4: Comparative long-term maternal and perinatal biological and psychosocial outcomes following VBAC, unsuccessful trial of labor, and elective repeat cesarean delivery are not well understood. We recommend well-designed studies to identify and describe these outcomes so adverse consequences can be mitigated or prevented.

Critical gap 5: The comparative effects that VBAC, unsuccessful trial of labor, and elective repeat cesarean delivery have on breastfeeding practices are not well understood. We recommend well-designed studies to identify these effects so adverse effects can be mitigated or prevented.

Critical gap 6: A variety of nonmedical factors affect the availability and management of trial of labor, but they have not been well studied. Access to safe trial of labor appears to be restricted by factors such as geography, workforce availability and training, professional association guidelines, type of maternity care provider, liability concerns, health insurance, and institutional policy. We recommend well-designed studies to better understand these factors and to test clinical, institutional, or policy interventions to increase access to safe trial of labor. Best practice models, such as those that incorporate risk stratification in forming policies for offering trial of labor and simulation training, should be developed and carefully assessed with an eye towards their widespread adoption.

Critical gap 7: The current medical-legal environment—including provider perceptions of and experience with professional liability—exerts a chilling effect on the availability of trial of labor. We recommend a series of clinical and policy-relevant studies to develop interventions to reduce this barrier.

Critical gap 8: The informed consent process for trial of labor and elective repeat cesarean delivery should be evidence-based, minimize bias, and incorporate a strong emphasis on the values and preferences of pregnant women. We recommend interprofessional collaboration to refine, validate, and implement decisionmaking and risk assessment tools, as well as informed consent templates that are informative and reliable, and that can be well documented. These tools should also communicate absolute risk in easily understood terms.

Critical gap 9: National and state-level surveillance of factors associated with trial of labor are lacking. We recommend that all states adopt the 2003 Standard Certificate of Live Birth and include questions in PRAMS about decisions regarding method of delivery, labor induction, and the role of the maternity care provider and mother (and partner) in the decisionmaking process from early pregnancy through delivery.

Critical gap 10: There is insufficient information on factors increasing VBAC among low-risk women. We recommend high-quality clinical studies of well-selected, low-risk women with sufficient statistical power to characterize risks for unsuccessful trial of labor in this population.

Conclusions

Given the available evidence, trial of labor is a reasonable option for many pregnant women with one prior low transverse uterine incision. The data reviewed in this report show that both trial of labor and elective repeat cesarean delivery for a pregnant woman with one prior transverse uterine incision have important risks and benefits and that these risks and benefits differ for the woman and her fetus. This poses a profound ethical dilemma for the woman as well as her caregivers, because benefit for the woman may come at the price of increased risk for the fetus and vice versa. This conundrum is worsened by the general paucity of high-level evidence about both medical and nonmedical factors, which prevents the precise quantification of risks and benefits that might help to make an informed decision about trial of labor compared with elective repeat cesarean delivery. We are mindful of these clinical and ethical uncertainties in making the following conclusions and recommendations.

One of our major goals is to support pregnant women with one prior transverse uterine incision to make informed decisions about trial of labor compared with elective repeat cesarean delivery. We recommend clinicians and other maternity care providers use the responses to the six questions, especially questions 3 and 4, to incorporate an evidence-based approach into the decisionmaking process. Information, including risk assessment, should be shared with the woman at a level and pace that she can understand. When trial of labor and elective repeat cesarean delivery are medically equivalent options, a shared decisionmaking process should be adopted and, whenever possible, the woman's preference should be honored.

We are concerned about the barriers that women face in gaining access to clinicians and facilities that are able and willing to offer trial of labor. Given the low level of evidence for the requirement for "immediately available" surgical and anesthesia personnel in current guidelines, we recommend that the American College of Obstetricians and Gynecologists and the American Society of Anesthesiologists reassess this requirement with specific reference to other obstetric complications of comparable risk, risk stratification, and in light of limited physician and nursing resources. Healthcare organizations, physicians, and other clinicians should consider making public their trial of labor policies and VBAC rates, as well as their plans for responding to obstetric emergencies. We recommend that hospitals, maternity care providers, healthcare and professional liability insurers, consumers, and policymakers collaborate on the development of integrated services that could mitigate or even eliminate current barriers to trial of labor.

We are concerned that medical-legal considerations add to, and in many instances exacerbate, these barriers to trial of labor. Policymakers, providers, and other stakeholders must collaborate in developing and implementating appropriate strategies to mitigate the chilling effect the medical-legal environment has on access to care.

High-quality research is needed in many areas. We have identified areas that need attention in response to question 6. Research in these areas should be given appropriate priority and should be adequately funded— especially studies that would help to characterize more precisely the short-term and long-term maternal, fetal, and neonatal outcomes of trial of labor and elective repeat cesarean delivery.

Consensus Development Panel

F. Gary Cunningham, M.D.
Panel and
  Conference Chairperson
Beatrice and Miguel Elias
  Distinguished Chair in
  Obstetrics and Gynecology
Professor
Department of Obstetrics and
  Gynecology
University of Texas Southwestern
  Medical Center at Dallas
Dallas, Texas

Shrikant I. Bangdiwala, Ph.D.
Professor
Department of Biostatistics,
  Research Track
Gillings School of Global
  Public Health
University of North Carolina
  at Chapel Hill
Chapel Hill, North Carolina

Sarah S. Brown, M.S.P.H.
Chief Executive Officer
The National Campaign
  to Prevent Teen and
  Unplanned Pregnancy
Washington, DC

Thomas Michael Dean, M.D.
Chief of Staff
Avera Weskota Memorial
  Medical Center
Staff Physician
Horizon Health Care, Inc.
Wessington Springs,
  South Dakota

Marilynn Frederiksen, M.D.
Associate Professor of Clinical
  Obstetrics and Gynecology
Feinberg School of Medicine
Northwestern University
Chicago, Illinois

Carol J. Rowland Hogue,
  Ph.D., M.P.H.
Jules & Uldeen Terry Professor
  of Maternal and Child Health
Professor of Epidemiology
Director
Women's and Children's Center
Rollins School of Public Health
Emory University
Atlanta, Georgia

Tekoa King, CNM, M.P.H., FACNM
Associate Clinical Professor
Department of Obstetrics,
  Gynecology, and
  Reproductive Sciences
University of California,
  San Francisco
Deputy Editor
Journal of Midwifery &
  Women's Health
San Francisco, California

Emily Spencer Lukacz, M.D., M.A.S.
Associate Professor
Clinical Reproductive Medicine
University of California,
  San Diego
La Jolla, California

35

Laurence B. McCullough, Ph.D.
*Dalton Tomlin Chair in Medical
   Ethics and Health Policy*
*Professor of Medicine and
   Medical Ethics*
Associate Director for Education
Center for Medical Ethics
   and Health Policy
Baylor College of Medicine
Houston, Texas

Wanda Nicholson, M.D., M.P.H.,
   M.B.A.
Associate Professor
Department of Obstetrics
   and Gynecology
University of North Carolina
   at Chapel Hill
Chapel Hill, North Carolina

Nancy Frances Petit, M.D.
*Chairperson, Division
   of Obstetrics*
St. Francis Hospital
Staff Obstetrician-Gynecologist
St. Francis OB/GYN Center
Newark, Delaware
Faculty
Uniformed Services University
   of Health Sciences
Bethesda, Maryland

Jeffrey Lynn Probstfield, M.D.
Adjunct Professor of Epidemiology
School of Public Health
Professor of Medicine (Cardiology)
Clinical Trials Service Unit
University of Washington
   School of Medicine
Seattle, Washington

Adele C. Viguera, M.D., M.P.H.
Associate Director
Perinatal and Reproductive
   Psychiatry Program
Neurological Institute
Cleveland Clinic
Cleveland, Ohio

Cynthia A. Wong, M.D.
Professor and Vice Chairperson
Chief of Obstetrical Anesthesia
Department of Anesthesiology
Northwestern University
Feinberg School of Medicine
Chicago, Illinois

Sheila Cohen Zimmet, R.N., J.D.
*Senior Associate Vice President
   for Regulatory Affairs*
Georgetown University
   Medical Center
Washington, DC

Speakers

David J. Birnbach, M.D., M.P.H.
Professor
Departments of Anesthesiology,
   Obstetrics and Gynecology,
   and Public Health
Executive Vice Chairman
Department of Anesthesiology
Associate Dean and Director
Center for Patient Safety
Miller School of Medicine
University of Miami
Miami, Florida

Emmanuel Bujold, M.D., M.Sc,
   FRCSC
Associate Professor
Maternal Fetal Medicine and
   Perinatal Epidemiology
*Jeanne et Jean-Louis Lévesque
   Research Chair*
Department of Obstetrics
   and Gynaecology
Faculty of Medicine
Laval University
Québec
CANADA

Karen B. Eden, Ph.D.
Investigator/Associate Professor
Department of Medical
  Informatics and Clinical
  Epidemiology
School of Medicine
Oregon Health and
  Science University
Portland, Oregon

Cathy Emeis, Ph.D., CNM
Investigator/Assistant Professor
Department of Primary Care
School of Nursing
Oregon Health and
  Science University
Portland, Oregon

Kimberly D. Gregory, M.D., M.P.H.
Vice Chairperson
Women's Healthcare Quality and
  Performance Improvement
Department of Obstetrics
  and Gynecology
Cedars-Sinai Medical Center
Los Angeles, California

William A. Grobman, M.D., M.B.A.
Associate Professor
Division of Maternal
  Fetal Medicine
Department of Obstetrics
  and Gynecology
Feinberg School of Medicine
Northwestern University
Chicago, Illinois

Jeanne-Marie Guise, M.D., M.P.H.
Principal Investigator/
  Associate Professor
Departments of Obstetrics
  and Gynecology, and
  Medical Informatics and
  Clinical Epidemiology
School of Medicine
Oregon Health and
  Science University
Portland, Oregon

Lucky Jain, M.D., M.B.A.
Richard W. Blumberg
  Professor and Executive
  Vice Chairperson
Department of Pediatrics
Emory University
  School of Medicine
Atlanta, Georgia

Miriam Kuppermann, Ph.D., M.P.H.
Professor
Departments of Obstetrics,
  Gynecology, & Reproductive
  Sciences, and Epidemiology
  & Biostatistics
University of California,
  San Francisco
San Francisco, California

Mark B. Landon, M.D.
Professor and Director
Division of Maternal-Fetal
  Medicine
Department of Obstetrics
  and Gynecology
The Ohio State University
  College of Medicine
Columbus, Ohio

Mona T. Lydon-Rochelle, Ph.D.,
  M.P.H., CNM
Associate Professor and
  Perinatal Epidemiologist
National Perinatal
  Epidemiology Centre
Anu Research Centre
Departments of Obstetrics
  and Gynaecology, and
  Epidemiology & Public Health
University College Cork
Cork University
  Maternity Hospital
Cork
IRELAND

Anne Drapkin Lyerly, M.D., M.A.
Associate Professor
Department of Obstetrics
    and Gynecology
Core Faculty
Trent Center for Bioethics,
    Humanities, and History
    of Medicine
Duke University
Durham, North Carolina

George A. Macones, M.D., M.S.C.E.
Professor and Chairperson
Department of Obstetrics
    and Gynecology
Washington University
    School of Medicine
St. Louis, Missouri

Howard Minkoff, M.D.
Distinguished Professor of
    Obstetrics and Gynecology
State University of New York–
    Downstate Medical Center
Chairperson
Department of Obstetrics
    and Gynecology
Maimonides Medical Center
Brooklyn, New York

T. Michael D. O'Shea, M.D., M.P.H.
Professor
Department of Pediatrics
Chief
Department of Neonatal
    & Perinatal Medicine
Neonatology Division
    of Pediatrics
School of Medicine
Wake Forest University
Winston-Salem, North Carolina

Rita Rubin
Medical Reporter
USA TODAY
McLean, Virginia

Caroline Signore, M.D., M.P.H.
Medical Officer
Pregnancy and
    Perinatology Branch
Eunice Kennedy Shriver
    National Institute of
    Child Health and
    Human Development
National Institutes of Health
Bethesda, Maryland

Robert M. Silver, M.D.
Professor and Chief
Division of Maternal-Fetal
    Medicine
Department of Obstetrics
    and Gynecology
University of Utah
    Health Sciences Center
Salt Lake City, Utah

Michael L. Socol, M.D.
Thomas J. Watkins
    Memorial Professor
    and Vice Chairperson
Department of Obstetrics
    and Gynecology
Division of Maternal-Fetal
    Medicine
Feinberg School of Medicine
Northwestern University
Chicago, Illinois

Chet Edward Wells, M.D.
Professor
Department of Obstetrics
    and Gynecology
University of Texas
    Southwestern Medical
    Center at Dallas
Dallas, Texas

Planning Committee

Duane Alexander, M.D.
*Planning Committee
  Chairperson*
Director
Eunice Kennedy Shriver Na-
  tional Institute
  of Child Health and Human
  Development
National Institutes of Health
Bethesda, Maryland

Caroline Signore, M.D., M.P.H.
*Planning Committee
  Chairperson*
Medical Officer
Pregnancy and
  Perinatology Branch
Eunice Kennedy Shriver
  National Institute of
  Child Health and
  Human Development
National Institutes of Health
Bethesda, Maryland

Lisa Ahramjian, M.S.
Communications Specialist
Office of Medical Applications
  of Research
Office of the Director
National Institutes of Health
Bethesda, Maryland

Shilpa Amin, M.D., M.Bsc., FAAFP
Medical Officer
Evidence-based Practice
  Centers Program
Center for Outcomes
  and Evidence
Agency for Healthcare
  Research and Quality
Rockville, Maryland

David J. Birnbach, M.D., M.P.H.
Professor
Departments of Anesthesiology,
  Obstetrics and Gynecology,
  and Public Health
Executive Vice Chairman
Department of Anesthesiology
Director
Center for Patient Safety
  and Associate Dean
Miller School of Medicine
University of Miami
Miami, Florida

Beth Collins Sharp, Ph.D., R.N.
Director
Evidence-based Practice
  Centers Program
Center for Outcomes
  and Evidence
Agency for Healthcare
  Research and Quality
Rockville, Maryland

Paul A. Cotton, Ph.D., R.D.
Program Director
Health Behavior and
  Minority Health
Division of Extramural Activities
National Institute of
  Nursing Research
National Institutes of Health
Bethesda, Maryland

F. Gary Cunningham, M.D.
*Panel and Conference
  Chairperson*
Beatrice and Miguel Elias
  Distinguished Chair in
  Obstetrics and Gynecology
Professor
Obstetrics and Gynecology
University of Texas Southwestern
  Medical Center at Dallas
Dallas, Texas

Planning Committee members provided their input at a meeting held
August 12–14, 2008. The information provided here was accurate at the
time of that meeting.

Lucky Jain, M.D., M.B.A.
Richard W. Blumberg Professor and Executive Vice Chairman
Department of Pediatrics
Emory University
  School of Medicine
Atlanta, Georgia

Luella Klein, M.D.
*Charles Howard
  Candler Professor*
Director
Regional Perinatal Center
Department of Gynecology
  and Obstetrics
Emory University
Atlanta, Georgia

Barnett S. Kramer, M.D., M.P.H.
*Associate Director for Disease
  Prevention*
Director
Office of Medical Applications
  of Research
Office of the Director
National Institutes of Health
Bethesda, Maryland

Mark B. Landon, M.D.
Professor
Director
Division of Maternal
  Fetal Medicine
Department of Obstetrics
  and Gynecology
The Ohio State University
  College of Medicine
Columbus, Ohio

Hal C. Lawrence, M.D.
Vice President
Practice Activities
American College
  of Obstetricians
  and Gynecologists
Washington, DC

Mona Theresa Lydon-Rochelle,
  Ph.D., M.P.H.
Clinical Associate Professor
Departments Global Health
  and Health Services
University of Washington
Bainbridge, Washington

George A. Macones, M.D., M.S.C.E.
Chairman
Department of Obstetrics
  and Gynecology
Washington University
  School of Medicine
St. Louis, Missouri

Kelli K. Marciel, M.A.
Communications Director
Office of Medical Applications
  of Research
Office of the Director
National Institutes of Health
Bethesda, Maryland

Howard Minkoff, M.D.
Professor
Department of Obstetrics
  and Gynecology
Maimonides Medical Center
SUNY-Brooklyn
Brooklyn, New York

Planning Committee members provided their input at a meeting held August 12–14, 2008. The information provided here was accurate at the time of that meeting.

Lata S. Nerurkar, Ph.D.
Senior Advisor for the Consensus
  Development Program
Office of Medical Applications
  of Research
Office of the Director
National Institutes of Health
Bethesda, Maryland

Judith P. Rooks, CNM, M.P.H., M.S.
American College
  of Nurse-Midwives
Portland, Oregon

Susan C. Rossi, Ph.D., M.P.H.
Deputy Director
Office of Medical Applications
  of Research
Office of the Director
National Institutes of Health
Bethesda, Maryland

James R. Scott, M.D.
Editor-In-Chief
Obstetrics and Gynecology
Professor and Chair Emeritus
Department of Obstetrics
  and Gynecology
University of Utah
  Medical Center
Salt Lake City, Utah

Robert M. Silver, M.D.
Professor
Division Chief of Maternal-Fetal
  Medicine
Department of Obstetrics
  and Gynecology
University of Utah
  Health Sciences Center
Salt Lake City, Utah

Catherine Y. Spong, M.D.
Chief
Pregnancy and
  Perinatology Branch
Eunice Kennedy Shriver
  National Institute of
  Child Health and
  Human Development
National Institutes of Health
Bethesda, Maryland

Linda J. Van Marter, M.D., M.P.H.
Associate Professor
  of Pediatrics
Harvard Medical School
Children's Hospital
Boston, Massachusetts

Planning Committee members provided their input at a meeting held
August 12–14, 2008. The information provided here was accurate at the
time of that meeting.

Conference Sponsors

Eunice Kennedy Shriver
  National Institute of
  Child Health and Human
  Development
Alan Guttmacher, M.D.
Acting Director

Office of Medical Applications
  of Research
Jennifer M. Croswell, M.D., M.P.H.
Acting Director

Conference Cosponsors

National Institute of
  Nursing Research
Patricia Grady, Ph.D., R.N.,
  FAAN
Director

Office of Research on
  Women's Health
Vivian W. Pinn, M.D.
*Associate Director for Research
  on Women's Health*

www.ingramcontent.com/pod-product-compliance
Lightning Source LLC
Chambersburg PA
CBHW051823170526
45167CB00005B/2134